Alessandro Benedetto

Icy Wellness

Discovering Well-Being through Ice Baths

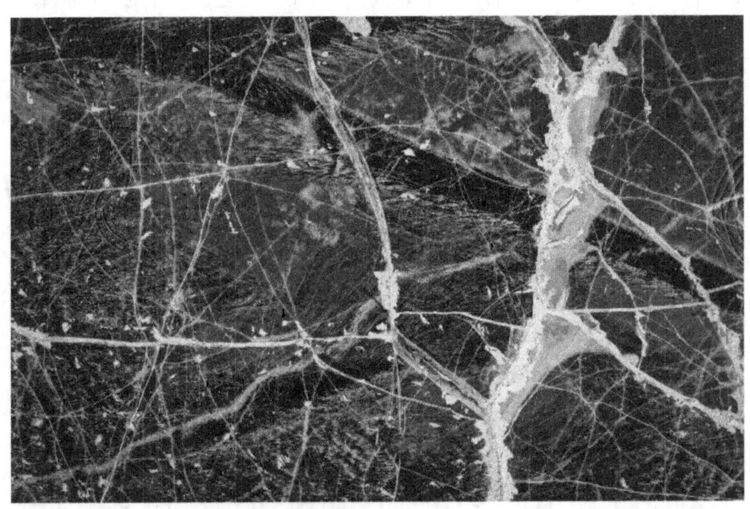

CHAPTER 1
INTRODUCTION

In a world where the pursuit of well-being has become a paramount goal, individuals are increasingly drawn to unconventional approaches that promise holistic benefits. One such practice that has emerged as both intriguing and transformative is the immersion in ice baths. This introduction sets the stage for a deep dive into the realm of icy wellness, exploring the profound impact that exposure to cold can have on our physical and mental health.

As we navigate through the pages that follow, we will uncover the therapeutic power embedded in the simplicity of cold water, discovering its potential to alleviate stress, improve sleep, boost energy levels, and enhance overall vitality. Beyond the contemporary fascination with ice baths, our journey will extend into the annals of history, tracing the roots of this practice across diverse cultures and civilizations.

This book is more than a mere endorsement of the benefits of ice baths; it is a comprehensive guide crafted to empower readers.

By blending scientific insights, practical guidance, and personal narratives, we aim to provide you with the tools and understanding necessary to embrace a lifestyle that incorporates the transformative effects of cold immersion. Welcome to a world where the chill of ice becomes a conduit to a renewed sense of well-being.

The Therapeutic Power of Cold

In the exploration of alternative methods for promoting well-being, one phenomenon gaining increasing recognition is the therapeutic potential inherent in exposure to cold. This chapter delves into the intricate ways in which cold temperatures can exert a profound impact on our physical and mental health, transcending the conventional boundaries of wellness practices.
Cold therapy, often harnessed through techniques like ice baths or cryotherapy, stimulates a cascade of physiological responses within the body. From vasoconstriction to the release of endorphins, the therapeutic journey into the cold introduces a repertoire of mechanisms that contribute to stress reduction, enhanced circulation, and immune system modulation.
As we unravel the therapeutic power of cold, we will navigate through the science underpinning these responses, exploring the intersection of ancient wisdom and modern research.

The chill of cold, it appears, is not merely an environmental condition but a potential catalyst for a holistic and rejuvenating approach to well-being.
Join us in deciphering the nuanced intricacies of this chilling yet invigorating expedition into the therapeutic realm of cold.

History of Ice Baths

The history of ice baths is a fascinating journey that spans diverse cultures and epochs, revealing a shared recognition of the invigorating and healing properties of cold water. From ancient civilizations to contemporary wellness practices, the tradition of immersing oneself in ice baths has evolved, leaving an indelible mark on the pursuit of physical and mental well-being.
Ancient civilizations, including the Greeks and Romans, were pioneers in recognizing the therapeutic benefits of cold water. Public bathhouses with cold plunge pools were integral to their communal spaces, offering a contrast to the warmth of traditional hot baths. The belief in the rejuvenating effects of cold water extended to cultures across Asia, where cold plunge pools and ice-cold rivers were embraced for their revitalizing properties.
Fast forward to the 19th century, and the use of cold water gained momentum as a therapeutic tool in Europe.

Hydrotherapy, which involved various water-based treatments, including cold baths, became a prominent aspect of medical practices. The work of figures like Vincent Priessnitz, a proponent of hydrotherapy, contributed to the popularization of cold water immersion for health benefits.

In more recent times, the resurgence of interest in ice baths can be traced to athletes and sports enthusiasts seeking effective recovery methods. The use of cold exposure for muscle recovery and inflammation reduction has become a staple in the training regimens of professional athletes worldwide.

As we explore the history of ice baths, it becomes evident that the allure of cold water transcends temporal and cultural boundaries, persisting as a timeless practice deeply intertwined with the human quest for well-being. This chapter unravels the rich tapestry of ice baths through the ages, shedding light on the enduring legacy of this age-old tradition.

Contemporary Revival and Innovation

While the historical roots of ice baths reveal a longstanding acknowledgment of their therapeutic benefits, the 21st century has witnessed a notable resurgence and innovative reinterpretation of this ancient practice. Modern science, coupled with a growing interest in holistic well-being, has propelled ice baths into the spotlight once again.

In recent decades, scientific research has delved into the physiological mechanisms underpinning the effects of cold exposure. Studies have explored how cold immersion impacts the cardiovascular system, triggers anti-inflammatory responses, and influences hormonal balance. This scientific validation has contributed to the integration of ice baths into wellness routines beyond traditional practices.

Moreover, technological advancements have played a pivotal role in transforming the way we experience ice baths. Cryotherapy chambers, equipped with controlled cold temperatures, offer a streamlined and efficient means of achieving the benefits associated with cold exposure. These innovations not only cater to athletes and fitness enthusiasts but also appeal to a broader audience seeking convenient and accessible methods for enhancing their well-being.

In the realm of sports, the adoption of ice baths as a recovery tool has become commonplace. Athletes, coaches, and sports science professionals recognize the potential of cold immersion in mitigating muscle soreness, expediting recovery between training sessions, and optimizing overall performance.

As we navigate through the chapters ahead, we will further explore how the history of ice baths intersects with contemporary practices. From ancient wisdom to cutting-edge technology, the journey of ice baths continues to evolve, promising new dimensions in the pursuit of well-being. Join us in unraveling the threads that connect the timeless tradition of cold immersion with the dynamic landscape of modern wellness.

Purpose of the Book

The purpose of this book is to serve as a comprehensive guide and source of inspiration for individuals seeking to explore and integrate the practice of ice baths into their lives. Beyond merely presenting the benefits of cold exposure, our aim is to empower readers with knowledge, practical insights, and a holistic understanding of how ice baths can contribute to overall well-being.

Inform and Educate:
This book endeavors to provide a thorough exploration of the therapeutic aspects of ice baths. By blending scientific explanations with historical contexts, we aim to inform readers about the physiological and psychological benefits associated with cold exposure.

Practical Guidance:
Recognizing that knowledge alone may not suffice, we offer practical advice on how to prepare for and engage in ice baths safely and effectively. From recommended durations and frequencies to variations in temperature and immersion methods, readers will find actionable guidance to tailor the practice to their preferences and needs.

Inspire Personal Exploration:
Through the sharing of personal anecdotes, success stories, and testimonials, we aspire to inspire readers to embark on their own journey of icy wellness. By illustrating the diverse ways in which individuals have integrated ice baths into their lives, we aim to ignite curiosity and encourage experimentation.

Bridge Ancient Wisdom with Modern Living:
Delving into the historical roots of ice baths, we aim to bridge the gap between ancient wisdom and contemporary lifestyles. The book explores how this age-old practice aligns with and complements modern approaches to well-being, offering a timeless yet adaptable tool for navigating the challenges of the present day.

Address Common Questions and Concerns: Recognizing that skepticism and questions may arise, we dedicate sections to address common concerns, misconceptions, and potential contraindications associated with ice baths. By offering transparent and evidence-based information, we aim to foster a deeper understanding of the practice.

Ultimately, the goal is to empower readers to make informed decisions about incorporating ice baths into their lives, fostering a sense of agency in their personal well-being journey. Whether you are a curious beginner or a seasoned enthusiast, this book strives to be a valuable companion in your exploration of the transformative world of icy wellness.

CHAPTER 2
Benefits of Ice Baths

Ice baths, with their invigorating chill, offer a multitude of benefits that extend beyond the immediate sensation of cold. As we explore the potential advantages of immersing oneself in icy waters, we uncover a range of physiological and psychological effects that contribute to overall well-being.

Stress Reduction:
Cold exposure prompts the release of
endorphins and activates the
parasympathetic nervous system, leading
to a state of relaxation. Ice baths can
serve as a powerful tool for stress
reduction, helping individuals manage the
demands of a hectic lifestyle and find
moments of tranquility.
Improved Sleep Quality:
The calming effect of cold exposure on the
nervous system can contribute to
improved sleep quality. By regulating the
sleep-wake cycle and promoting
relaxation, ice baths may be particularly
beneficial for those seeking a natural and
non-pharmaceutical approach to sleep
enhancement.
Increased Energy and Alertness:
Cold immersion stimulates the release of
adrenaline and noradrenaline, leading to
heightened alertness and increased
energy levels. Many individuals report a
sense of rejuvenation and mental clarity
after an ice bath, making it a potential
strategy for boosting daytime vitality.
Enhanced Circulation:
The vasoconstrictive and vasodilatory
effects of cold exposure contribute to
improved circulation.

This can be particularly advantageous for individuals looking to support cardiovascular health and promote efficient blood flow throughout the body.

Benefits for Skin and Muscle Recovery:
Cold exposure is known to reduce inflammation, making ice baths a popular choice for athletes and fitness enthusiasts seeking faster muscle recovery. Additionally, the constriction of blood vessels during cold immersion can tighten pores and promote healthier skin.

Immune System Modulation:
Cold exposure has been linked to positive effects on the immune system. While excessive stress on the body can suppress immune function, controlled exposure to cold may enhance the body's resilience and immune response.

These benefits, among others, contribute to the growing appeal of ice baths as a holistic wellness practice. Whether used as a recovery tool, a stress management strategy, or a means of promoting overall vitality, the potential advantages of embracing the cold are varied and compelling. In the chapters ahead, we will delve deeper into the science behind these benefits and explore how individuals from different walks of life have incorporated ice baths into their well-being routines.

Stress Reduction

In the relentless pace of modern life, stress
has become an omnipresent force that can
profoundly impact both our physical and
mental well-being. Ice baths, with their
unique ability to induce a physiological
response to cold, emerge as a compelling
ally in the quest for stress reduction.
Cold exposure prompts the release of
endorphins, the body's natural feel-good
chemicals. These neurotransmitters
interact with receptors in the brain,
creating a sense of euphoria and acting as
a natural stress reliever.
Immersing oneself in icy waters stimulates
the parasympathetic nervous system, often
referred to as the "rest and digest" system.
This activation counterbalances the "fight
or flight" response associated with stress,
inducing a state of relaxation and calm.
Exposure to cold has been linked to the
modulation of cortisol, a hormone released
in response to stress. Ice baths may
contribute to regulating cortisol levels,
potentially mitigating the detrimental
effects of chronic stress on the body.
The relaxation induced by cold exposure
extends to its potential to improve sleep
quality.

By calming the nervous system, ice baths create an environment conducive to restful sleep, offering respite from the mental strain associated with stress.
The intentional act of engaging in an ice bath fosters mindfulness, encouraging individuals to be present in the moment. This mindfulness practice can contribute to stress awareness, allowing individuals to develop healthier coping mechanisms for managing stressors in their lives.

As we explore the role of ice baths in stress reduction, we uncover a multifaceted approach that combines physiological responses with mindfulness, offering individuals a holistic strategy to navigate the challenges of stress in their daily lives. In the subsequent chapters, we will delve deeper into the science behind these stress-relieving effects and provide practical guidance for incorporating ice baths into stress management routines.

Improvement of Sleep Quality

In the pursuit of enhanced well-being, the quest for better sleep is often paramount. Ice baths, with their unique influence on the body's physiological responses, present an intriguing avenue for those seeking to improve the quality of their sleep.

Exposure to cold has been associated with the regulation of the circadian rhythm, the body's internal clock that governs the sleep-wake cycle. Ice baths may contribute to aligning this cycle, promoting a more consistent and restorative pattern of sleep. The calming effect of cold exposure extends to the nervous system, triggering the activation of the parasympathetic nervous system. This relaxation response can counteract the heightened states of arousal or stress that often interfere with falling asleep and maintaining restful sleep. Cooling the body through an ice bath induces a drop in core body temperature. This decline in temperature mimics the natural drop that occurs before sleep onset, signaling to the body that it is time to rest. This temperature-induced sleepiness can facilitate a smoother transition into sleep. Ice baths may offer benefits for individuals experiencing symptoms of insomnia. The relaxation and endorphin release associated with cold exposure can alleviate anxiety and tension, common contributors to sleep disturbances.

For those grappling with sleep deprivation, ice baths can serve as a rejuvenating tool.

The release of endorphins and the overall calming effect may provide a natural boost in energy, aiding individuals in navigating the challenges of the day after a night of compromised sleep.

As we delve into the realm of sleep improvement through ice baths, it becomes evident that the potential benefits extend beyond the physiological realm into the intricacies of sleep psychology. The chapters that follow will further illuminate these aspects and offer practical insights for incorporating ice baths into a personalized sleep enhancement routine.

Increased Energy

In the perpetual quest for sustained vitality and heightened productivity, the potential of ice baths to boost energy levels emerges as a captivating facet of their holistic benefits. The invigorating effects of cold exposure extend beyond a mere wake-up call, offering a nuanced approach to enhancing overall energy and alertness.
The exposure to cold prompts the release of adrenaline, a hormone that plays a key role in the "fight or flight" response. This surge in adrenaline provides a natural energy boost, promoting alertness and heightened cognitive function.

Cold immersion also stimulates the release of noradrenaline, a neurotransmitter associated with arousal and attentiveness. The combined action of adrenaline and noradrenaline creates a synergistic effect, contributing to increased mental clarity and focus.

The drop in core body temperature induced by cold exposure triggers the body to expend energy in order to maintain its normal temperature. This process, known as thermogenesis, can result in a temporary metabolic boost, potentially enhancing overall energy levels.

The release of endorphins during and after an ice bath contributes to an improved mood, fostering a positive outlook and heightened motivation. This uplift in mood can translate into increased energy for daily activities and challenges.

Ice baths, particularly when used as a recovery tool after physical exertion, can alleviate muscle fatigue and reduce feelings of lethargy. The overall sense of physical rejuvenation contributes to a more energized state, enhancing one's ability to tackle tasks with vigor.

As we explore the synergy between cold exposure and increased energy, it becomes clear that ice baths offer a dynamic approach to revitalizing both the body and mind. The ensuing chapters will further illuminate the science behind these energy-boosting effects and provide practical guidance for individuals looking to incorporate ice baths into their routines for sustained vitality.

Benefits for Skin and Circulation

The benefits of ice baths extend beyond internal physiological responses to encompass external effects on the skin and the circulatory system. The invigorating chill of cold immersion brings about a range of positive outcomes, contributing to both the health and appearance of the skin while influencing overall circulatory function.

Cold exposure induces vasoconstriction followed by vasodilation, a process that exercises the blood vessels and promotes enhanced circulation. This heightened blood flow can contribute to better oxygenation of tissues and improved nutrient delivery throughout the body.

Cold immersion is renowned for its anti-inflammatory effects. By constricting blood vessels, ice baths can alleviate inflammation, making them a popular choice for individuals seeking relief from conditions such as sore muscles, joint pain, and swelling.

The contrast between the cold water and the body's natural temperature can promote a healthier complexion. Cold exposure tightens pores, reduces puffiness, and may contribute to an improved skin tone and texture.
Regular ice baths are often lauded for their potential to enhance the skin's natural radiance.
As a recovery tool, ice baths aid in reducing muscle soreness and fatigue. The improved circulation resulting from cold exposure facilitates the removal of metabolic byproducts, helping muscles recover more efficiently after physical exertion.
The anti-inflammatory properties of cold immersion may have positive implications for individuals dealing with certain skin conditions, such as eczema or psoriasis.
While individual responses can vary, some may find relief through the calming effects of cold exposure.
Cold exposure has been associated with enhanced cellular repair processes. The stress response induced by cold immersion can trigger mechanisms that promote cellular renewal, contributing to overall skin health.

As we navigate through the interconnected benefits for skin and circulation, it becomes evident that the impact of ice baths extends beyond the immediate sensation of cold.

The subsequent chapters will delve into the underlying science and practical considerations related to harnessing these benefits for a comprehensive approach to well-being.

Impact on the Immune System

The relationship between ice baths and the immune system is a compelling aspect of their potential health benefits. While cold exposure is known to elicit stress responses in the body, it also engages mechanisms that can contribute to the modulation and strengthening of the immune system.
The stress response induced by cold exposure is a form of hormesis—an adaptive response to a moderate stressor that results in enhanced resilience. This hormetic effect may extend to the immune system, stimulating beneficial adaptations that contribute to improved immune function.
Cold exposure has been associated with an increase in the activity of certain white blood cells, such as granulocytes and monocytes. These immune cells play a crucial role in the body's defense against pathogens, suggesting that ice baths may support a more robust immune response.
Chronic inflammation can compromise immune function. The anti-inflammatory properties of cold immersion may help mitigate excessive inflammation, creating an environment that supports a balanced immune response.

Cold exposure activates brown adipose tissue, leading to the production of heat. This process, known as thermogenesis, may have implications for immune function, as BAT is thought to play a role in metabolic and immune regulation.

Cold exposure has been shown to influence the production of cytokines, signaling proteins that regulate immune responses. The modulation of cytokine activity may contribute to a fine-tuned and effective immune system.

Regular exposure to cold may foster adaptation and resilience within the immune system. By challenging the body in a controlled manner, ice baths may contribute to the development of a more responsive and adaptable immune system.

Understanding the nuanced interplay between cold exposure and immune function provides insights into the potential of ice baths as a holistic wellness practice. As we explore the scientific foundations of this relationship, subsequent chapters will offer practical guidance on leveraging ice baths to support immune health in a balanced and intentional manner.

CHAPTER 3
The Science Behind Cold Exposure

The physiological responses triggered by exposure to cold form a fascinating intersection of ancient wisdom, modern research, and the intricate workings of the human body. This chapter aims to unravel the science behind cold exposure, shedding light on the complex mechanisms that underlie the transformative effects of immersing oneself in icy waters.

When the body is exposed to cold, blood vessels initially constrict (vasoconstriction) to conserve heat. This is followed by vasodilation, where the blood vessels expand. This cycle exercises the vascular system, promoting improved circulation and delivering essential nutrients throughout the body.

Cold exposure prompts the release of endorphins, the body's natural painkillers and mood elevators. These neurotransmitters interact with receptors in the brain, creating a sense of euphoria and contributing to the overall well-being associated with cold immersion.

The shock of cold triggers the release of adrenaline and noradrenaline, hormones associated with the "fight or flight" response. This hormonal surge induces heightened alertness, increased energy levels, and an overall state of heightened physiological readiness.

Cold exposure activates brown adipose tissue (BAT), a type of fat that generates heat when metabolized. This process, known as thermogenesis, contributes to the body's ability to maintain a stable core temperature and may have implications for metabolic health.

Cold exposure influences the release of various hormones, including cortisol. While acute stressors can elevate cortisol levels, controlled exposure to cold may contribute to hormonal balance over time, potentially mitigating the negative effects of chronic stress.

Cold immersion is associated with a reduction in inflammation, which can have broad implications for health. The anti-inflammatory response may contribute to faster recovery from exercise-induced muscle damage and provide relief for individuals dealing with inflammatory conditions.

Cold exposure has been linked to mitochondrial biogenesis—the creation of new mitochondria, the energy powerhouses of cells. This process enhances cellular energy production and may contribute to increased endurance and overall vitality.

Understanding the intricate dance between cold exposure and the body's responses opens the door to a deeper appreciation of the potential benefits associated with this practice. As we delve into the scientific nuances, the subsequent chapters will explore how these physiological mechanisms translate into tangible improvements in well-being and offer practical guidance for incorporating cold exposure into a holistic lifestyle.

Physiological Response to Cold

The human body's intricate response to cold is a finely tuned orchestra of physiological mechanisms designed to maintain core temperature and adapt to environmental challenges. Understanding this response provides insights into the transformative effects of cold exposure on various bodily systems.
When exposed to cold, blood vessels near the skin's surface constrict (vasoconstriction) to minimize heat loss. This initial response is a crucial adaptive mechanism that conserves warmth and redirects blood flow to vital internal organs.
Cold exposure activates brown adipose tissue (BAT), a unique type of fat that generates heat through thermogenesis. BAT activation contributes to the body's ability to produce warmth and plays a role in regulating overall metabolic activity.

In response to cold, the body may initiate shivering—a rapid, involuntary muscle contraction. Shivering generates heat as a byproduct of muscle activity, helping to elevate core body temperature.

Cold exposure triggers the release of endorphins, the body's natural mood enhancers and pain relievers. This endorphin release contributes to the exhilarating and euphoric sensations often associated with activities like ice baths.

The shock of cold prompts the release of adrenaline and noradrenaline, hormones associated with the "fight or flight" response. This hormonal surge leads to increased heart rate, heightened alertness, and mobilization of energy resources.

Cold exposure influences the secretion of various hormones, including cortisol. While acute stressors can elevate cortisol levels, controlled exposure to cold may contribute to hormonal balance over time, potentially influencing stress resilience.

Cold exposure, particularly through cryotherapy, is associated with a reduction in inflammation. This anti-inflammatory effect has implications for recovery from exercise-induced muscle damage and may offer relief for individuals dealing with inflammatory conditions.

Cold exposure can lead to an elevation in metabolic rate as the body works to produce heat. This increase in energy expenditure may contribute to weight management and improved metabolic function.

Understanding the body's intricate physiological response to cold unveils the complexity of these adaptive mechanisms. The subsequent chapters will delve deeper into how these responses translate into tangible benefits for well-being and provide practical insights for individuals looking to leverage the transformative power of cold exposure.

Effects on Inflammation

The relationship between cold exposure and inflammation is a multifaceted interplay that extends beyond the immediate sensation of cold. Understanding how cold influences the inflammatory response provides insights into its potential therapeutic applications and benefits.
Cold exposure has been associated with a decrease in inflammatory markers. This includes a reduction in pro-inflammatory cytokines and other molecules that contribute to the inflammatory response. The dampening of these markers may have implications for individuals dealing with chronic inflammatory conditions.

The body's response to cold may engage anti-inflammatory pathways. This modulation of the immune response contributes to a balanced inflammatory state, promoting a more controlled and efficient reaction to stressors.

Cryotherapy, a form of cold therapy, is often utilized to reduce inflammation and promote healing. By constricting blood vessels and minimizing blood flow to affected areas, cryotherapy may alleviate swelling and enhance the recovery process, particularly after injuries or intense physical activity.

Athletes frequently turn to cold exposure, such as ice baths, to aid in muscle recovery. Cold helps mitigate exercise-induced muscle damage by reducing inflammation and promoting efficient removal of metabolic byproducts associated with tissue stress.

In certain situations, the anti-inflammatory effects of cold exposure may contribute to pain relief. Cold numbs nerve endings and reduces the transmission of pain signals, making it a popular choice for managing acute pain or discomfort.

Controlled exposure to cold may contribute to a balance in the body's inflammatory responses. Rather than suppressing the immune system, this balance ensures that inflammation serves its protective functions without becoming chronic or detrimental to overall health.

Cold therapy is often employed for joint health, especially in conditions like arthritis. The reduction in inflammation around joints can lead to decreased pain and improved mobility, offering individuals a non-pharmaceutical approach to managing joint-related discomfort.

Understanding how cold exposure impacts inflammation provides a foundation for considering its application in various health contexts. In the subsequent chapters, we will delve into specific scenarios where cold exposure may be beneficial in managing inflammation and offer practical insights for incorporating these practices into a well-rounded wellness routine.

Role of Hormones in Thermal Stress

The interaction between the body and thermal stress involves a complex hormonal response, orchestrating a series of physiological changes to adapt and maintain internal balance. Understanding the role of hormones in thermal stress provides insights into how the body navigates and responds to changes in temperature.

Cortisol, often referred to as the stress hormone, plays a crucial role in the body's response to thermal stress.

Exposure to cold or heat can influence cortisol levels, with cold exposure potentially leading to an initial increase in cortisol release.

This hormone helps regulate energy metabolism and contributes to the body's ability to adapt to stressors.

Thermal stress, especially in the form of cold exposure, triggers the release of adrenaline and noradrenaline from the adrenal glands. These hormones initiate the "fight or flight" response, elevating heart rate, increasing alertness, and mobilizing energy reserves to cope with the stressor.

Exposure to extreme temperatures can impact thyroid hormone levels, influencing metabolic rate. In colder conditions, the body may increase thyroid hormone production to generate more heat through increased metabolism. Conversely, in hotter conditions, thyroid activity may decrease to conserve energy.

Thermal stress, particularly cold exposure, has been associated with the release of growth hormone. This hormone plays a role in cellular repair, regeneration, and overall growth, contributing to the body's adaptive response to stress.

Thermal stress, whether from cold or heat, can influence the release of vasopressin, an antidiuretic hormone. Vasopressin helps regulate fluid balance by affecting water reabsorption in the kidneys, aiding the body in adapting to temperature-induced changes in hydration needs.

Thermal stress may impact sex hormone production, although the specific effects can vary. Research suggests that factors such as cold exposure may influence sex hormone levels, potentially playing a role in the body's adaptation to environmental stressors.

Thermal stress, particularly cold exposure, prompts the release of endorphins—natural opioids that contribute to pain relief and mood elevation. This hormonal response is part of the body's adaptive mechanism to mitigate the discomfort associated with extreme temperatures.

Understanding the orchestration of these hormones during thermal stress provides a holistic view of the body's intricate response to environmental challenges. The subsequent chapters will delve into how these hormonal changes translate into physiological adaptations and discuss practical considerations for incorporating thermal stress into wellness routines.

Chapter 4
How to Prepare for and Practice Ice Baths

Embracing ice baths as part of your wellness routine requires thoughtful preparation and a mindful approach to the practice. Whether you're a beginner or an experienced enthusiast, here's a comprehensive guide on how to prepare for and effectively practice ice baths.

Before incorporating ice baths into your routine, especially if you have pre-existing health conditions, it's advisable to consult with a healthcare professional. They can provide personalized advice based on your individual health status.
If you're new to ice baths, start gradually to allow your body to acclimate. Begin with shorter durations and milder temperatures, progressively increasing as you become more comfortable with the experience.
Select a suitable location for your ice bath. If using a bathtub, ensure it's clean and free from any sharp objects. If using an outdoor source, ensure it's safe and free from contaminants.

Gather Necessary Supplies:
Ice or ice packs
Thermometer to monitor water temperature
Towels for drying off
Warm clothing for post-immersion
Optional: timer to track immersion duration

Drink plenty of water before your ice bath to ensure you're well-hydrated. Hydration is essential for supporting the body's response to cold stress.
Engage in light physical activity or take a warm shower before the ice bath. This helps increase blood flow and prepares your body for the cold exposure.
When entering the ice bath, do so slowly and mindfully. Focus on your breath and try to relax your body. Consider submerging one body part at a time to ease into the cold.
Practice controlled breathing during the ice bath. Deep, slow breaths can help manage the initial shock of the cold and promote relaxation.
Pay attention to how your body responds. If you experience discomfort beyond a manageable level, exit the ice bath. It's essential to prioritize safety and individual comfort.
After the ice bath, gently dry off and change into warm clothing. Focus on maintaining a comfortable body temperature as your body continues to adapt.

As you become more accustomed to ice baths, consider gradually increasing immersion time or experimenting with colder temperatures. Listen to your body and progress at a pace that feels right for you.
Support your body's recovery with activities such as light movement, stretching, or a warm beverage. Pay attention to how your body feels in the hours following the ice bath.
Consistent practice allows your body to adapt and maximize the potential benefits of ice baths. Find a frequency that suits your schedule and aligns with your overall wellness goals.

Remember, individual responses to ice baths can vary, so it's essential to customize the experience based on your comfort level and health considerations. Always prioritize safety, and if in doubt, seek guidance from a healthcare professional or experienced practitioner.

Safety Tips for Ice Baths

Embracing the practice of ice baths comes with numerous benefits, but it's crucial to prioritize safety to ensure a positive and secure experience.

Here are essential safety tips to consider before, during, and after your ice bath sessions:

Before the Ice Bath:

Before incorporating ice baths into your routine, especially if you have existing health conditions or concerns, consult with a healthcare professional for personalized advice.
Be aware of any medical conditions or medications that may contradict cold exposure. Individuals with conditions such as Raynaud's disease or cardiovascular issues should exercise caution and seek guidance.
If you're new to ice baths, start with short durations and milder temperatures. Allow your body to acclimate gradually to minimize the risk of shock.
Stay well-hydrated before your ice bath session. Proper hydration supports your body's ability to respond to cold stress.

During the Ice Bath:

If possible, have someone nearby to supervise or assist you during the ice bath, especially if you're new to the practice.
Enter the ice bath slowly and mindfully. Consider submerging one body part at a time to help your body adjust to the cold gradually.

Practice controlled breathing to manage the initial shock of the cold. Deep, slow breaths can promote relaxation and help you adapt to the temperature.
Be mindful of the duration of your ice bath. Start with shorter sessions and gradually increase as your body becomes more accustomed to the cold.

After the Ice Bath:

After the ice bath, warm up your body gradually. Engage in light physical activity or take a warm shower to restore your core temperature.
Change into warm clothing promptly after the ice bath to maintain a comfortable body temperature. Layering is a good practice to retain warmth.
Pay attention to how your body responds to each ice bath session. If you experience prolonged discomfort or adverse effects, adjust the duration or temperature accordingly.

General Safety Considerations:

Prolonged exposure to extreme cold can lead to conditions like hypothermia. Avoid extended periods in the ice bath, especially if you're new to the practice.

If you experience severe discomfort, numbness, or pain beyond a manageable level, exit the ice bath immediately. Prioritize your well-being and safety.

Periodically reassess your health status and consult with a healthcare professional. Factors such as changes in health conditions or medications may impact your suitability for ice baths.

Consistent practice is beneficial, but always exercise caution and listen to your body. What works for one person may not be suitable for another.

By incorporating these safety tips into your ice bath routine, you can enjoy the benefits of this practice while prioritizing your well-being. Remember that individual responses vary, and it's essential to customize your approach based on your comfort level and health considerations.

Recommended Duration and Frequency

Determining the optimal duration and frequency of ice baths is a nuanced process that depends on individual factors, health considerations, and personal goals. Here are general guidelines to help you navigate the duration and frequency of ice bath sessions:

Duration:

Begin with shorter durations, such as 5 to 10 minutes, especially if you are new to ice baths. Allow your body to acclimate to the cold gradually.
As your body becomes accustomed to the practice, you can gradually increase the duration. Aim for a maximum duration of 15 to 20 minutes per session, but always prioritize comfort and safety.
Pay attention to how your body responds. If you experience prolonged discomfort, numbness, or shivering beyond a manageable level, it may be an indication to shorten the duration.
The purpose of your ice bath may influence the ideal duration. For recovery after intense physical activity, shorter sessions may be effective. If you're seeking the potential benefits of cold exposure for stress reduction, longer sessions may be explored with caution.

Frequency:

Consistency in ice bath practice contributes to the body's adaptation and potential benefits. Aim for regular sessions, such as 2 to 3 times per week, to establish a routine.

Pay attention to how your body responds between sessions. If you experience any signs of prolonged stiffness, discomfort, or unusual fatigue, consider adjusting the frequency.

The frequency of ice baths can vary based on your goals. Athletes engaged in intense training may benefit from more frequent sessions, while individuals using ice baths for stress reduction might find benefit in fewer, longer sessions. Consider your individual recovery needs. Factors such as the intensity and frequency of your physical activities, overall health, and lifestyle play a role in determining the ideal frequency of ice baths.

Safety and Adaptation:

If you have pre-existing health conditions or concerns, consult with healthcare professionals, physiotherapists, or experienced practitioners to tailor the duration and frequency of ice baths to your specific needs.

As your body adapts to cold exposure, you may find that you can comfortably extend both the duration and frequency. However, always prioritize safety and avoid pushing beyond your limits.

Remember that individual responses to ice baths can vary, and it's essential to customize the duration and frequency based on your comfort level, health status, and goals. Regular reassessment and, if necessary, consultation with professionals will contribute to a safe and effective ice bath practice.

Variations in Temperature and Immersion Methods

The practice of ice baths encompasses a spectrum of temperatures and immersion methods, each offering unique benefits and considerations. Understanding these variations allows individuals to tailor their approach based on personal preferences, tolerance levels, and specific wellness objectives.

Temperature Variations:
Moderate Cold (10-15°C / 50-59°F):

Description: A mild introduction to cold exposure.
Benefits: Enhances circulation, supports recovery after physical activity, and stimulates a mild stress response.
Considerations: Suitable for beginners or those easing into cold exposure.

Cold (5-10°C / 41-50°F):

Description: A more intense cold experience with noticeable effects.
Benefits: Amplifies circulation, promotes anti-inflammatory responses, and may enhance mental alertness.
Considerations: Gradual acclimatization is crucial; listen to your body's signals.

Very Cold (0-5°C / 32-41°F):

Description: Intense cold exposure with pronounced physiological responses.
Benefits: Potentially boosts metabolism, increases endorphin release, and enhances stress resilience.
Considerations: Reserved for experienced individuals; closely monitor your body's reactions.

Extreme Cold (< 0°C / < 32°F):

Description: Extreme cold with significant challenges.
Benefits: Intensive stress response, potential for heightened alertness, and robust physiological adaptation.
Considerations: Advanced practitioners only; prioritize safety and gradual progression.

Immersion Methods:

Full Immersion:

Description: Entire body submersion in cold water, typically in a bathtub or natural water source.
Benefits: Comprehensive cold exposure, engaging the entire body for systemic effects.
Considerations: Ensure proper supervision, especially for beginners; monitor body temperature.

Partial Immersion:

Description: Immersing specific body parts, such as legs or arms, in cold water.
Benefits: Targeted exposure for localized benefits, often used for targeted recovery.
Considerations: Easier to control for beginners; adjust based on individual comfort.

Contrast Bathing (Hot-Cold Alternation):

Description: Alternating between hot and cold water immersion.
Benefits: Enhances circulation, may reduce muscle soreness, and provides a dynamic contrast for the body.

Considerations: Requires access to both hot and cold water sources; adapt ratios based on preference.

Cryotherapy Chambers or Cubicles:

Description: Enclosed spaces with controlled cold temperatures.
Benefits: Efficient and controlled exposure, often used in professional settings.
Considerations: Professional guidance recommended; potential for intense cold.

Understanding the spectrum of temperature variations and immersion methods allows individuals to tailor their ice bath practice to align with personal goals and comfort levels. Whether opting for a mild introduction or embracing extreme cold exposure, safety, gradual progression, and attentive self-monitoring remain paramount.

Enhancing your ice bath experience goes beyond the cold water itself. Incorporating the right tools and accessories can contribute to comfort, safety, and an overall positive immersion. Here are key items to consider for a well-rounded ice bath experience:

Thermometer:
Purpose: Monitor water temperature accurately.
Benefits: Ensures the water temperature aligns with your preferences and safety guidelines.

Ice or Ice Packs:
Purpose: Regulate and control water temperature.
Benefits: Enables you to adjust the coldness of the water based on your comfort level and desired intensity.

Timer:
Purpose: Track immersion duration.
Benefits: Helps you manage and gradually increase exposure time, ensuring a mindful practice.

Towels:
Purpose: Dry off post-immersion.
Benefits: Essential for warmth and comfort after exiting the ice bath; consider using a warm towel for added coziness.

Warm Clothing:
Purpose: Retain body heat after the ice bath.
Benefits: Prevents rapid heat loss, especially in colder environments; layering is effective for insulation.

Anti-Slip Mat or Bath Mat:
Purpose: Enhance safety during entry and exit.
Benefits: Provides stability, reducing the risk of slipping on wet surfaces.

Floatation Device:
Purpose: Aid in buoyancy and relaxation.
Benefits: Especially useful in natural water sources; enhances comfort and eases tension.

Music or Meditation App:
Purpose: Facilitate relaxation and mindfulness.
Benefits: Creates a soothing atmosphere; music or guided meditations can enhance the mental aspect of the experience.

Hot Water Source (for Contrast Bathing):
Purpose: Alternate between hot and cold immersion.

Benefits: Adds a dynamic contrast, potentially enhancing circulation and recovery.

Cryotherapy Chambers or Cubicles:
Purpose: Controlled cold exposure.
Benefits: Offers a streamlined and efficient experience; commonly used in professional settings.

Sauna or Hot Tub (for Contrast Bathing):
Purpose: Alternating between hot and cold environments.
Benefits: Expands the contrast effect, potentially amplifying circulation benefits; provides a diverse thermal experience.

Aromatherapy Diffuser:
Purpose: Infuse the environment with pleasant scents.
Benefits: Enhances the sensory experience; select calming scents for relaxation.

Comfortable Seating or Stool:
Purpose: Facilitate a relaxed position during immersion.
Benefits: Useful for prolonged sessions; ensures comfort and stability.

First Aid Kit:
Purpose: Address minor injuries or discomfort.
Benefits: Essential for immediate care; include items like bandages, antiseptic wipes, and pain relief medication.

Health Monitoring Devices:
Purpose: Track vital signs.
Benefits: For advanced practitioners, devices like heart rate monitors can provide insights into physiological responses.

Customizing your ice bath experience with these tools and accessories allows you to create a personalized, safe, and enjoyable routine. Always prioritize safety and gradual progression, and adapt your tools based on individual preferences and goals.

Specially Designed Tubs and Containers

Investing in purpose-built tubs and containers can elevate the ice bath experience, providing comfort, safety, and convenience. Here are considerations for tubs and containers specifically designed for cold exposure:

Ice Bath Tubs:
Dedicated containers designed for cold immersion.
Insulated walls to retain cold temperature.

Slip-resistant surfaces for safety.
Comfortable seating or contours for
ergonomic support.
Options for various sizes to accommodate
individual preferences.

Portable Ice Baths:
Convenient solutions for on-the-go or
outdoor use.
Lightweight and collapsible for easy
transport.
Durable materials for outdoor settings.
Quick-drain systems for efficient post-
immersion handling.
Insulation to maintain cold temperature.

Inflatable Ice Baths:
Space-saving and versatile cold
immersion options.
Inflatable design for easy setup and
storage.
Soft and comfortable interior.
Options with built-in seats for added
comfort.
Sturdy construction for durability.

Wooden Ice Tubs:
Aesthetically pleasing and durable
immersion containers.
Insulating properties of wood.
Rustic or contemporary designs to suit
preferences.

Varying sizes for solo or group use.
Sealed and treated wood for longevity.

Hydrotherapy Tubs:
Designed for a combination of hot and cold water
therapy.
Adjustable temperature settings.
Jets for hydrotherapy massage.
Ergonomic design for comfort.
Options with in-built heating and cooling
systems.

Customizable Containers:
Personalized solutions tailored to individual
needs.
Options for insulation customization.
Adjustability for water depth and temperature.
Compatibility with accessories like seats and
covers.
Durable and easy-to-clean materials.

Medical-Grade Ice Baths:
Designed for professional and therapeutic use.
Precise temperature control.
Options for water circulation.
Hygienic and easy-to-clean surfaces.
Compliant with medical standards.

Outdoor Ice Pools:
Larger containers for group or recreational use.
Options for both cold and contrast bathing.
Sturdy construction for outdoor use.
Customization for landscaping integration.
Seating and safety features for group settings.

Choosing a tub or container with features that align with your preferences and intended use ensures a more enjoyable and effective ice bath experience. Whether prioritizing portability, aesthetics, or therapeutic functionality, purpose-built containers provide a foundation for a personalized and comfortable practice.

Supplements and Recovery Products

Incorporating supplements and specialized recovery products into your routine can enhance the effectiveness of post-exercise recovery. Here are considerations for various supplements and products designed to support recovery:

Protein Powders: Aid muscle repair and growth.

Benefits: Convenient source of high-quality protein.
Rapid absorption for post-workout recovery.
Varied types include whey, casein, and plant-based options.

BCAAs (Branched-Chain Amino Acids): Support muscle protein synthesis and reduce muscle soreness.
Leucine, isoleucine, and valine promote recovery.
Ideal for workouts with high intensity or volume.
Available in powder or capsule form.

Creatine: Enhance strength, power, and muscle recovery.
Supports ATP regeneration for energy.
Aids in muscle cell hydration.
Particularly beneficial for high-intensity activities.

Electrolyte Drinks: Replenish electrolytes lost through sweat.
Prevents dehydration and muscle cramping.
Ideal for intense or prolonged exercise.
Contains minerals like sodium, potassium, and magnesium.

Omega-3 Fatty Acids: Combat inflammation and support joint health.
Omega-3s contribute to reduced muscle soreness.
Support overall cardiovascular health.

Found in fish oil supplements or algae-based options for vegetarians.

Turmeric or Curcumin Supplements: Natural anti-inflammatory properties.
Alleviates exercise-induced inflammation.
Supports joint health.
Often combined with black pepper (piperine) for enhanced absorption.

Collagen Supplements: Support connective tissue health.
Aids in tendon and ligament recovery.
Supports skin, hair, and nail health.
Available in powder, capsule, or liquid form.

Compression Gear: Enhance circulation and reduce muscle soreness.
Supports muscle recovery through compression.
Improves blood flow and reduces swelling.
Various garments include socks, sleeves, and full-body suits.

Foam Rollers and Massage Tools: Self-myofascial release and muscle relaxation.
Reduces muscle tightness and soreness.
Improves flexibility and range of motion.
Various tools include foam rollers, massage sticks, and massage balls.

When incorporating supplements and recovery products, it's important to consider individual needs, dietary restrictions, and potential interactions with other medications. Consulting with a healthcare professional or a nutritionist can provide personalized guidance based on specific health considerations and fitness goals.

Chapter 6

Success Stories and Testimonials

Hearing the experiences of individuals who have embraced ice baths and cold exposure can provide inspiration and valuable insights. Here are some success stories and testimonials from individuals who have incorporated cold exposure into their wellness routines:

Sarah's Recovery Journey:
Sarah, a dedicated athlete, discovered the power of ice baths for recovery after intense training sessions. She shares how incorporating regular cold exposure has significantly reduced post-workout muscle soreness and improved her overall performance. Sarah emphasizes the importance of gradual adaptation and how the mental resilience gained from ice baths positively influences her training mindset.

Mark's Stress Reduction Success:
Mark, a high-stress professional, found solace in the practice of cold exposure for stress reduction. Through consistent ice baths, Mark shares how he has experienced a profound improvement in his ability to manage stress, increased mental clarity, and enhanced focus. Mark's journey underscores the holistic benefits of cold exposure beyond physical recovery.

Emily's Journey to Better Sleep:
Struggling with sleep disturbances, Emily explored various methods for improving her sleep quality. She recounts how incorporating cold exposure into her evening routine has positively impacted her sleep patterns. Emily emphasizes the calming effect of ice baths on her nervous system, leading to more restful and rejuvenating nights.

John's Weight Loss Transformation:
John embarked on a weight loss journey that included a holistic approach to health. He shares how cold exposure became a valuable tool in his weight loss strategy.

Regular cold showers and ice baths, combined with a healthy lifestyle, contributed to John's successful weight loss, increased metabolism, and improved overall well-being.

Jessica's Mental Resilience Boost:
Jessica, a busy professional balancing work and family life, highlights the mental benefits she gained from incorporating cold exposure. She describes how the practice has become a form of mindfulness, helping her stay present and focused amid life's challenges. Jessica credits ice baths for cultivating mental resilience and enhancing her overall mental well-being.

Mike's Joint Health Improvement:
Dealing with joint discomfort, Mike turned to cold exposure as a natural remedy. He shares how cold therapy, including contrast baths and localized applications, has provided relief for his joint issues. Mike emphasizes the importance of consistency and gradual progression in realizing the long-term benefits for joint health.

Anna's Immune System Support:
Anna, who faced frequent bouts of illness, incorporated cold exposure into her routine to strengthen her immune system.

She describes how the practice of cold showers and ice baths has reduced the frequency of illnesses and enhanced her overall immune resilience. Anna encourages others to explore the immune-boosting potential of cold exposure.

These success stories and testimonials showcase the diverse ways in which individuals have integrated cold exposure into their lives, realizing benefits that extend beyond physical recovery. Whether seeking mental clarity, stress reduction, improved sleep, or specific health goals, these accounts highlight the versatility and transformative potential of cold exposure practices.

Impact on Various Aspects of Life

Embracing cold exposure can have a multifaceted impact on different dimensions of an individual's life, encompassing physical well-being, mental resilience, and overall lifestyle. Here are insights into how cold exposure practices influence various aspects of life:

Physical Resilience and Recovery:
Cold exposure, such as ice baths and contrast bathing, can contribute to enhanced physical resilience. Individuals often report reduced muscle soreness, improved recovery after intense exercise, and increased tolerance to cold conditions.
Mental Clarity and Focus:
Cold exposure is linked to heightened mental alertness and clarity. Many practitioners describe a sense of invigoration and increased focus after exposure to cold, attributing it to the release of endorphins and improved circulation to the brain.
Stress Reduction and Emotional Well-being:
Cold exposure serves as a unique stress management tool. Regular practices, like cold showers or plunges, are associated with the activation of the body's stress response, leading to an increased ability to cope with stressors. This, in turn, contributes to improved emotional well-being.
Quality of Sleep:
Incorporating cold exposure into one's routine has been reported to positively influence sleep patterns. The calming effect of cold on the nervous system may contribute to more restful and rejuvenating sleep, leading to improved overall sleep quality.
Immune System Support:
Exposure to cold is believed to stimulate the immune system.

Many individuals who practice cold exposure report a reduction in the frequency and severity of illnesses, attributing it to the potential immune-boosting effects of cold exposure.

Community and Social Connection: Cold exposure, especially in group settings or social events, fosters a sense of community and connection. Shared experiences during ice baths or cold plunges often create a supportive environment, where individuals encourage each other to push boundaries and explore the benefits of cold exposure together.

Mindfulness and Mental Toughness: Engaging in cold exposure requires a level of mindfulness and mental toughness. Practitioners often find that the discipline required to face the discomfort of the cold contributes to increased mental resilience, encouraging a positive mindset in the face of challenges.

Lifestyle Integration and Adaptation:
Cold exposure practices can become integral parts of individuals' lifestyles. Whether it's incorporating cold showers into daily routines or scheduling regular ice baths, these practices often lead to lifestyle adaptations. Over time, individuals develop a greater appreciation for the adaptability and resilience of their bodies.

Environmental Appreciation:
Cold exposure practices often instill a newfound appreciation for the environment. Whether immersing in natural bodies of water or simply embracing the cold outdoors, individuals develop a heightened connection to nature and its elements.

These insights into the impact of cold exposure underscore its potential to positively influence various aspects of life. From physical resilience and mental clarity to social connection and lifestyle integration, cold exposure practices offer a holistic approach to well-being.

Chapter 7
Ice Baths and Sports Performance

The integration of ice baths into athletes' training regimens has gained popularity for its potential impact on sports performance and recovery. Here's a look at how ice baths influence different aspects of athletic performance:

Ice baths are known to be effective in mitigating muscle soreness and inflammation following intense physical activity. The cold temperature helps constrict blood vessels, reducing blood flow to the affected muscles. Subsequent rewarming may promote improved circulation, aiding in the removal of metabolic waste and reducing inflammation.

Athletes often engage in multiple training sessions in a day or week. Ice baths can accelerate recovery between sessions by minimizing muscle damage and inflammation. This allows athletes to maintain a higher training frequency and intensity, contributing to overall performance improvements.

Ice baths can contribute to enhanced muscle and joint function.

The reduction in muscle soreness and inflammation may lead to improved flexibility and joint range of motion, crucial for athletes in various sports.

Athletes often face challenges in regulating body temperature during intense training. Ice baths act as a form of thermal stress, training the body to adapt to temperature fluctuations. This adaptation may enhance an athlete's ability to manage heat stress during competition.

The discomfort associated with cold exposure in ice baths can contribute to mental toughness. Athletes who regularly undergo cold exposure may develop increased resilience to physical discomfort, potentially translating into improved focus and mental strength during competition.

For athletes training in hot climates, ice baths can serve as a pre-emptive measure against heat-related issues. The adaptation to cold stress may improve an athlete's tolerance to high temperatures, reducing the risk of heat-related conditions during competition.

Ice baths have shown benefits for athletes engaged in endurance sports. By reducing muscle soreness and inflammation, athletes may recover more quickly between long-duration sessions, allowing for sustained high-performance levels over time.

While ice baths offer potential benefits for sports performance and recovery, it's important to note that individual responses may vary. Athletes should consider consulting with sports science professionals or healthcare providers to tailor ice bath strategies to their specific needs and training regimens.

Muscle Recovery and Inflammation Reduction

Cold exposure, particularly through practices like ice baths, plays a crucial role in muscle recovery and the reduction of inflammation for individuals engaged in physical activities. Here's an exploration of how these cold exposure methods contribute to these key aspects:

Cold exposure, such as immersion in ice baths, is effective in mitigating muscle soreness post-exercise. The cold temperature helps constrict blood vessels, reducing swelling and inflammation in the muscles. This contributes to a quicker recovery process.

Intense physical activity often induces inflammation in the muscles due to micro-tears and oxidative stress.

Cold exposure has been shown to reduce this exercise-induced inflammation by limiting the release of pro-inflammatory substances. This reduction in inflammation is vital for overall muscle health.

Cold exposure enhances the recovery process by facilitating muscle repair. The constriction and subsequent dilation of blood vessels encourage the removal of metabolic waste products and the delivery of oxygen and nutrients to the muscles. This promotes the repair of damaged muscle fibers.

Ice baths are commonly employed to prevent or alleviate Delayed Onset Muscle Soreness (DOMS), which often occurs after strenuous or unaccustomed exercise. Cold exposure helps minimize the severity of DOMS by addressing the inflammatory response and reducing muscle damage.

Athletes and fitness enthusiasts often incorporate ice baths into their recovery routines to optimize the overall recovery time between training sessions. This is particularly beneficial for those engaging in high-frequency or high-intensity training, allowing for more consistent performance.

Cold exposure contributes to improved flexibility and range of motion in muscles and joints.

By reducing inflammation and promoting better blood flow, individuals may experience enhanced mobility, crucial for preventing injuries and maintaining optimal performance.

The vasoconstriction and vasodilation triggered by cold exposure contribute to improved blood circulation. This enhanced circulation helps flush out metabolic byproducts from muscle tissues and ensures a more efficient supply of nutrients and oxygen, vital for recovery. Cold exposure aids in the reduction of swelling and edema in injured or stressed muscles. This anti-swelling effect is particularly relevant in the context of acute injuries or conditions requiring immediate attention.

Incorporating cold exposure methods for muscle recovery and inflammation reduction is a well-established practice in the realms of sports and fitness. While the benefits are significant, it's important for individuals to tailor their cold exposure practices based on their unique requirements and preferences.

Practical Applications for Athletes and Fitness Enthusiasts

The integration of cold exposure into the routines of athletes and fitness enthusiasts offers a range of practical applications that contribute to enhanced performance, recovery, and overall well-being.

Athletes often utilize post-exercise ice baths to accelerate recovery. Submerging the body in cold water, typically ranging from 10 to 15 degrees Celsius (50 to 59 degrees Fahrenheit), helps reduce muscle soreness, inflammation, and facilitates faster recovery between training sessions.

Incorporating cold showers into daily routines provides a convenient and accessible form of cold exposure. Cold showers contribute to muscle recovery, stimulate circulation, and offer an energy-boosting effect. Many individuals choose to end their regular shower with a brief burst of cold water.

Contrast bathing involves alternating between hot and cold water immersion. This practice enhances circulation, with the cold phase helping to constrict blood vessels and reduce inflammation, while the hot phase promotes relaxation. This method is effective in improving blood flow and reducing muscle soreness.

For acute injuries or localized pain, applying ice packs or cold compresses can be beneficial. Localized cold therapy helps reduce swelling, numbs the affected area, and alleviates pain. This is commonly employed in the treatment of injuries like sprains, strains, or minor bruises. Some athletes incorporate whole-body cryotherapy, which involves exposure to extremely cold temperatures for a short duration, as part of their pre-competition routine.

While research on its efficacy is ongoing, some athletes report feeling invigorated and mentally prepared after cryotherapy sessions.

Ice massage involves applying ice directly to a specific area using circular motions. This technique is useful for targeting small muscle groups or areas prone to tension. Ice massage can aid in reducing localized inflammation and promoting recovery.

Endurance athletes, such as marathon runners or cyclists, often use cold water immersion to address the demands of their training. Immersing legs in cold water post-endurance exercise can help alleviate muscle fatigue and reduce the risk of overuse injuries.

Athletes preparing for competitions in hot climates may use cold exposure to aid in heat acclimatization. By adapting to cold stress, individuals may improve their ability to regulate body temperature and tolerate heat during events.

Incorporating these practical applications of cold exposure requires an understanding of individual preferences, fitness goals, and specific needs.

Athletes and fitness enthusiasts may experiment with various methods to tailor their cold exposure practices, ensuring a safe and effective integration into their overall training regimens. It's advisable to consult with healthcare or fitness professionals to create a personalized approach that aligns with individual goals and well-being.

Chapter 8
Ice Baths in the Context of Traditional Medicine

While ice baths and cold exposure practices are often associated with modern wellness and sports science, various traditional medicine systems have recognized the therapeutic benefits of exposure to cold. Here's an exploration of how ice baths align with principles found in certain traditional medicinal practices:
Traditional Chinese Medicine, rooted in the concept of balancing vital energies (Qi), acknowledges the importance of temperature balance for overall health. Cold exposure, when approached mindfully, is seen as a way to balance the body's energies. Ice baths may be considered to help regulate Qi and promote harmony within the body.

Ayurveda, the ancient Indian system of medicine, emphasizes the balance of bodily doshas (Vata, Pitta, Kapha). Contrast therapies, involving alternating hot and cold elements, are a part of Ayurvedic practices.

Ice baths align with the principles of contrast therapy, contributing to a dynamic balance of doshas and supporting overall well-being.

In Nordic and Scandinavian cultures, exposure to cold through practices like ice swimming has deep historical roots. These traditions have long recognized the invigorating effects of cold water on both physical and mental health. Cold exposure in this context is often viewed as a natural and integral part of a healthy lifestyle.

Russian Banya (sauna) traditions frequently involve cycles of intense heat followed by a plunge into cold water or snow. This contrast is believed to purify the body and stimulate circulation. The cold exposure component is seen as an essential element for achieving holistic health benefits.

Japanese bathing culture, as seen in traditional public baths (Sento) and hot springs (Onsen), involves the contrast of hot and cold elements. Cold plunge pools or outdoor cold baths are common features, believed to promote circulation, relieve muscle tension, and invigorate the body.
Certain Native American tribes incorporate sweat lodge ceremonies that involve cycles of heat and cold.

While not directly equivalent to ice baths, these ceremonies recognize the purifying effects of temperature variations, aligning with the idea of balancing the body's energies.
Hydrotherapy, a form of traditional medicine widely practiced in Europe, includes the use of water in various temperatures for therapeutic purposes. Cold water applications, such as cold plunges or dousing, are believed to stimulate the circulatory and immune systems.
Winter traditions in Baltic and Eastern European cultures often involve cold exposure, such as rolling in the snow after a sauna session. These practices are rooted in the belief that exposure to cold enhances vitality, strengthens the immune system, and promotes overall health.

While the terminology and specific practices may vary, the fundamental idea of using cold exposure for therapeutic purposes is a thread that runs through diverse traditional medicine systems. Ice baths, when approached with respect for individual constitutions and conditions, align with these historical practices, reflecting a cross-cultural acknowledgment of the potential benefits of cold exposure for health and well-being.

Integrated Approaches to Health

In the pursuit of holistic well-being, contemporary health practices increasingly recognize the significance of integrated approaches that address the interconnectedness of physical, mental, and emotional aspects of health. Here's an exploration of key components within integrated approaches to health: Integrated health embraces a holistic paradigm, acknowledging that optimal well-being goes beyond the absence of illness. It considers physical, mental, emotional, and social dimensions, emphasizing the interconnectedness of these elements in achieving a state of holistic wellness.

Integrated health recognizes the profound connection between the mind and the body. Practices such as mindfulness, meditation, and yoga are integral components that foster mental well-being while influencing physical health. The mind-body connection underscores the impact of mental states on physiological functions.
Nutrition is a cornerstone of integrated health. It goes beyond conventional dietary recommendations and emphasizes the role of food as medicine. Nutritional medicine focuses on individualized dietary plans, nutrient-dense foods, and the prevention and management of health conditions through proper nutrition.
Integrated health incorporates various complementary and alternative modalities alongside conventional medical practices. Modalities such as acupuncture, herbal medicine, chiropractic care, and traditional healing practices contribute to a diverse toolkit for personalized health interventions.
Physical activity is considered a vital aspect of integrated health. Exercise not only contributes to physical fitness but also has profound effects on mental and emotional well-being. Integrated approaches emphasize the importance of incorporating diverse forms of movement suitable for individual preferences and health goals.

Integrated health recognizes the impact of the environment on overall well-being. This includes aspects such as clean air, water, and sustainable living practices. Environmental health considerations extend to creating living and working environments that support optimal health outcomes.

Integrated health places a strong emphasis on preventive care and lifestyle modifications. Lifestyle medicine interventions, including stress management, adequate sleep, and behavioral changes, aim to prevent and manage chronic conditions by addressing root causes and promoting healthier habits.

Mental health is a central focus within integrated approaches. Psychosocial support services, counseling, and mental health interventions are integrated seamlessly with physical health care. This acknowledges the significance of mental well-being in achieving overall health goals.

Integrated approaches to health recognize that well-being is a dynamic interplay of various factors.

By fostering collaboration between conventional and complementary practices and addressing the multifaceted nature of health, these approaches aim to empower individuals to take an active role in their overall well-being.

Therapeutic Support for Specific Disorders

In the realm of healthcare, therapeutic interventions tailored to specific disorders play a crucial role in addressing and managing various health conditions. Here's an overview of therapeutic support for specific disorders:

Cognitive-Behavioral Therapy (CBT) for Anxiety Disorders:
CBT is widely employed to treat anxiety disorders, such as generalized anxiety disorder, panic disorder, and social anxiety. It focuses on identifying and challenging negative thought patterns, promoting behavioral changes, and developing coping strategies to alleviate anxiety symptoms.
Medication Management for Depressive Disorders:
Depressive disorders often involve a combination of psychotherapy and medication management. Antidepressant medications, such as selective serotonin reuptake inhibitors (SSRIs) or serotonin-norepinephrine reuptake inhibitors (SNRIs), are commonly prescribed alongside therapy to address symptoms of depression.

Applied Behavior Analysis (ABA) for Autism Spectrum Disorder (ASD):
ABA is an evidence-based therapeutic approach used for individuals with Autism Spectrum Disorder. It focuses on assessing and modifying behaviors, teaching new skills, and fostering social interaction. ABA interventions are often tailored to the unique needs of individuals with ASD.
Dialectical Behavior Therapy (DBT) for Borderline Personality Disorder:
DBT is specifically designed for individuals with Borderline Personality Disorder (BPD). It combines cognitive-behavioral techniques with mindfulness practices. DBT aims to help individuals regulate emotions, improve interpersonal skills, and develop effective coping mechanisms.
Speech-Language Therapy for Communication Disorders:
Speech-language therapy is essential for individuals with communication disorders, including speech and language delays, stuttering, or aphasia. Therapists work to enhance communication skills, improve articulation, and address language difficulties based on the specific disorder.
Occupational Therapy for Sensory Processing Disorder (SPD):

Occupational therapy is beneficial for individuals with Sensory Processing Disorder (SPD). Therapists use sensory integration techniques to help individuals better process and respond to sensory information, improving daily functioning and behavior.

Exposure Therapy for Phobias and Post-Traumatic Stress Disorder (PTSD):

Exposure therapy is commonly used to treat phobias and PTSD. It involves gradually and safely exposing individuals to feared situations or traumatic memories, allowing them to confront and process the associated anxiety or trauma in a controlled therapeutic environment.

Antipsychotic Medications for Schizophrenia:

Antipsychotic medications are often prescribed for individuals diagnosed with schizophrenia. These medications help alleviate symptoms such as hallucinations and delusions, allowing individuals to better engage in therapy and manage their condition.

These therapeutic interventions exemplify the diversity of approaches employed in healthcare to address specific disorders. The selection of therapeutic modalities depends on the nature of the disorder, individual preferences, and the collaborative efforts of healthcare professionals to ensure comprehensive and tailored support for each individual.

Who Can Benefit from Ice Baths?

Ice baths, with their potential therapeutic effects, can be beneficial for a variety of individuals across different lifestyles and health conditions. Here's an overview of who might derive benefits from ice baths:

Athletes and Sports Enthusiasts:
Benefit: Ice baths are commonly used by athletes post-exercise to aid in muscle recovery, reduce inflammation, and manage muscle soreness. They can be particularly beneficial for those engaging in high-intensity training and competitive sports.
Fitness Enthusiasts:
Benefit: Individuals who participate in regular fitness routines, including weightlifting, high-intensity interval training (HIIT), or endurance exercises, may find ice baths helpful in minimizing exercise-induced muscle damage and promoting faster recovery.

Rehabilitation and Injury Recovery:
Benefit: People undergoing rehabilitation for injuries, such as strains or sprains, may benefit from ice baths to manage inflammation and facilitate the recovery process.
Cold exposure can assist in reducing pain and swelling associated with injuries.
Chronic Pain and Inflammatory Conditions:
Benefit: Individuals dealing with chronic pain conditions or inflammatory disorders, such as arthritis, may find relief through ice baths. The cold temperature can help alleviate inflammation and provide temporary pain relief.
Stress Management:
Benefit: Ice baths may contribute to stress management by inducing a "cold stress" response, which can have positive effects on the nervous system. The discomfort associated with cold exposure may trigger a stress adaptation response, potentially improving resilience to stressors.
Improvement of Sleep Quality:
Benefit: Ice baths have been associated with improvements in sleep quality. The cooling effect on the body may contribute to the regulation of circadian rhythms, helping individuals achieve better sleep patterns.

Enhanced Circulation and Cardiovascular Health:
Benefit: Cold exposure in ice baths can promote vasoconstriction and vasodilation, leading to improved blood circulation. This can have positive effects on cardiovascular health, potentially supporting heart function and overall circulatory well-being.
Mood and Mental Well-Being:
Benefit: Cold exposure is linked to the release of endorphins, the body's natural "feel-good" chemicals. Ice baths may contribute to an improved mood and mental well-being, offering a refreshing and invigorating experience.
It's important to note that individual responses to ice baths can vary, and certain populations, such as pregnant individuals or those with certain medical conditions, should consult with healthcare professionals before incorporating ice baths into their routines. Additionally, personalized approaches, including consideration of individual tolerance and preferences, are key to optimizing the benefits of ice baths.

Possible Contraindications and Precautions

While ice baths can offer various benefits, it's crucial to be aware of potential contraindications and take necessary precautions. Here are considerations for individuals considering or currently practicing ice baths:
Cardiovascular Conditions:
Precaution: Individuals with cardiovascular conditions, such as heart disease or hypertension, should exercise caution with cold exposure. Extreme cold can lead to increased heart rate and blood pressure, potentially exacerbating cardiovascular issues. Consultation with a healthcare professional is advised.
Respiratory Conditions:
Precaution: People with respiratory conditions, including asthma or chronic obstructive pulmonary disease (COPD), may find cold air challenging to breathe. Cold exposure could potentially trigger respiratory symptoms, so individuals with such conditions should be cautious and consult with a healthcare provider.
Pregnancy:
Precaution: Pregnant individuals should approach cold exposure with care. Extreme cold may lead to vasoconstriction, affecting blood flow, and could potentially impact the developing fetus. Consultation with a healthcare provider is essential to ensure the safety of both the parent and the baby.

Raynaud's Disease:
Contraindication: Individuals with Raynaud's disease, a condition characterized by restricted blood flow to certain parts of the body, may be more sensitive to cold temperatures. Ice baths can exacerbate symptoms and are generally contraindicated. Consultation with a healthcare professional is advised.
Open Wounds or Infections:
Precaution: It's important to avoid cold exposure if there are open wounds, cuts, or infections on the skin. Cold temperatures can impair the body's natural healing process and may increase the risk of complications. Wait until the skin has fully healed before engaging in ice baths.
Neurological Conditions:
Precaution: Individuals with certain neurological conditions, such as neuropathy or multiple sclerosis, may have altered sensations in extremities. Extreme cold can exacerbate these sensations and may not be suitable. Consultation with a healthcare provider is recommended.
Individual Tolerance:

Precaution: Cold tolerance varies among individuals. It's important to pay attention to personal comfort levels during ice baths. Prolonged exposure or excessively cold temperatures may lead to discomfort, shivering, or, in extreme cases, hypothermia. Gradual adaptation and monitoring are advised.
Age Considerations:
Precaution: Children and older adults may have different responses to cold exposure. Care should be taken to ensure that the experience is comfortable and safe for individuals in these age groups. Consultation with healthcare professionals is recommended, especially for older adults.
In all cases, individuals considering ice baths or cold exposure practices should seek guidance from healthcare professionals, especially if they have pre-existing health conditions or concerns. Tailoring cold exposure to individual needs and tolerances is crucial for a safe and positive experience.

Responses to Common Doubts and Skepticisms

When introducing new concepts, such as ice baths, individuals may have doubts or express skepticism. Here are responses to address common doubts and concerns:

Doubt: "Are ice baths safe?"
Response: Ice baths are generally safe when practiced responsibly. It's crucial to start with shorter durations and gradually increase exposure based on individual tolerance. If you have underlying health conditions, consult with a healthcare professional before incorporating ice baths into your routine.
Doubt: "I heard cold exposure is uncomfortable. Why would anyone willingly do it?"
Response: While cold exposure can be initially uncomfortable, many individuals find it invigorating and enjoy the benefits it offers, such as improved recovery, stress reduction, and increased energy. The discomfort often becomes more manageable with regular practice.
Skepticism: "Do ice baths really help with muscle recovery?"
Response: Yes, ice baths can contribute to muscle recovery by reducing inflammation and minimizing muscle soreness. The cold exposure helps constrict blood vessels, flushing out waste products and promoting faster healing. Many athletes and fitness enthusiasts incorporate ice baths into their recovery routines.

Skepticism: "Is there scientific evidence supporting the benefits of ice baths?"
Response: Yes, scientific studies suggest that ice baths can have positive effects on recovery, inflammation, and overall well-being. While more research is ongoing, there is evidence supporting the therapeutic potential of cold exposure. Individual responses may vary.
Doubt: "Won't I just get used to the cold, and it won't be effective anymore?"
Response: The body can adapt to cold exposure to some extent, but the benefits can still be maintained. It's important to vary the duration and temperature of ice baths to prevent complete adaptation. Additionally, incorporating other recovery strategies can enhance overall effectiveness.
Doubt: "I'm not an athlete. Can I still benefit from ice baths?"
Response: Absolutely. Ice baths are not exclusive to athletes. They can benefit individuals from various backgrounds by promoting overall well-being, reducing stress, and improving circulation. Consider starting with shorter durations and adapting the practice to your comfort level.

Skepticism: "I've heard cold exposure is bad for the immune system. Is that true?"
Response: While extreme cold exposure can temporarily suppress the immune system, moderate cold exposure, such as ice baths, is generally considered safe and may even have immune-supportive effects. As with any health practice, individual factors should be considered, and consultation with healthcare professionals is advised.

Doubt: "I'm concerned about the potential for hypothermia. How can I avoid that?"
Response: Hypothermia is a valid concern. To avoid it, start with shorter ice bath durations, gradually increasing exposure. Monitor your body's response, and avoid prolonged exposure in extremely cold temperatures. Always prioritize safety and consult with healthcare professionals if you have concerns.
When addressing doubts or skepticism, providing clear and informed responses helps individuals make informed decisions about whether ice baths are suitable for them. Encourage an open dialogue and suggest seeking guidance from healthcare professionals for personalized advice.

Chapter 10
Conclusions

In conclusion, the practice of ice baths emerges as a multifaceted approach to well-being, offering a range of potential benefits for individuals across diverse lifestyles. Through a historical exploration, we unveiled the roots of cold exposure practices, showcasing their presence in various cultures and traditional healing systems.

Delving into the therapeutic realm, we navigated through the potential physiological and psychological impacts of ice baths. From stress reduction and enhanced sleep to immune system support and athletic recovery, the evidence suggests a broad spectrum of positive outcomes associated with embracing the cold.

The journey continued with a comprehensive examination of factors such as safety, contraindications, and precautions.

Recognizing that individual responses may vary, we emphasized the importance of tailored approaches, encouraging individuals to listen to their bodies and seek professional guidance when needed.

Furthermore, the integration of ice baths into the broader context of holistic health and well-being was explored.

From the mind-body connection to the principles of integrated health, we illuminated how this practice aligns with comprehensive approaches to fostering vitality and balance.

As we navigated through responses to common doubts and skepticism, we highlighted the importance of open-minded exploration and personal adaptation. Ice baths, while not a one-size-fits-all solution, offer a dynamic space for individuals to discover their own thresholds and preferences.

In the spirit of well-rounded exploration, the journey touched upon the potential for cultural integration and the intersection of ice baths with traditional healing practices. From the wisdom of Traditional Chinese Medicine to Nordic traditions and beyond, the practice finds resonance across a rich tapestry of cultural landscapes.

In the final analysis, the path forward involves a nuanced consideration of personal goals, health conditions, and individual preferences. Ice baths stand as an invitation to explore the invigorating realms of cold exposure, promoting resilience, recovery, and a sense of vitality.

In the realm of well-being, as in the practice of ice baths, the journey is as important as the destination. It is a journey that calls for self-awareness, adaptability, and an appreciation for the diverse ways in which individuals can cultivate their own paths to optimal health.

May the exploration of ice baths, with its rich tapestry of history, science, and cultural significance, inspire individuals to embark on their own journeys toward well-being, resilience, and the discovery of the extraordinary potential within the embrace of the cold.

s we conclude this exploration into the world of ice baths and their potential impact on well-being, I extend an invitation for you to embark on your own personal journey of discovery. The practice of ice baths, with its rich historical roots and diverse therapeutic possibilities, invites individuals to explore the realms of cold exposure in a way that aligns with their unique aspirations and wellness goals.

Here are a few considerations as you venture into your personal exploration:

Start with Curiosity:

Allow curiosity to guide your exploration. Approach the practice of ice baths with an open mind, acknowledging the potential benefits while remaining attuned to your own comfort levels and preferences.

Listen to Your Body:
Your body is a remarkable guide. Pay attention to how it responds to cold exposure. If discomfort turns into pain or if you experience unusual sensations, it's essential to listen and adjust accordingly. Respect your body's signals.
Gradual Adaptation:
Like any new practice, gradual adaptation is key. Begin with shorter durations and less extreme temperatures. As your body becomes accustomed, you can progressively increase exposure. This allows for a safer and more comfortable experience.
Consultation with Professionals:
If you have pre-existing health conditions or concerns, consider consulting with healthcare professionals before incorporating ice baths into your routine. Their guidance can provide personalized insights based on your individual health status.
Embrace Individual Preferences:

Ice baths are a versatile practice that can be adapted to suit individual preferences. Experiment with variations in temperature, duration, and frequency to find what resonates best with you. Personalizing the experience enhances its effectiveness and enjoyment.

Combine with Holistic Wellness Practices:
Consider integrating ice baths into a broader framework of holistic wellness. Combine this practice with other elements such as mindfulness, healthy nutrition, and regular exercise to create a comprehensive approach to well-being.

Explore Cultural Perspectives:
Dive into the cultural perspectives surrounding cold exposure. Explore how various traditions and healing systems view the benefits of embracing the cold. Understanding the cultural context adds depth to your exploration.

Share Experiences and Learnings:
Engage in conversations with others who have explored or are exploring ice baths. Share your experiences and learnings. The collective wisdom of a community can offer insights and diverse perspectives.

Stay Open to Adaptation:
Your wellness journey is dynamic. Stay open to adapting your approach based on how your body responds and evolves.

Embrace the flexibility to modify your practice in alignment with your changing needs.
As you embark on this journey, may it be a source of empowerment, self-discovery, and enhanced well-being. Ice baths offer a unique avenue for personal exploration, and your individual path holds the potential for resilience, vitality, and a deeper connection with your own extraordinary capacity for wellness. Enjoy the adventure!

www.ingramcontent.com/pod-product-compliance
Lightning Source LLC
Chambersburg PA
CBHW060957260726
48661CB00005B/1921